BLOOD TYPE

O COOKBOOK

"60+ Nutritious and Delicious Recipes for your Blood Type to Help with Optimal Wellness"

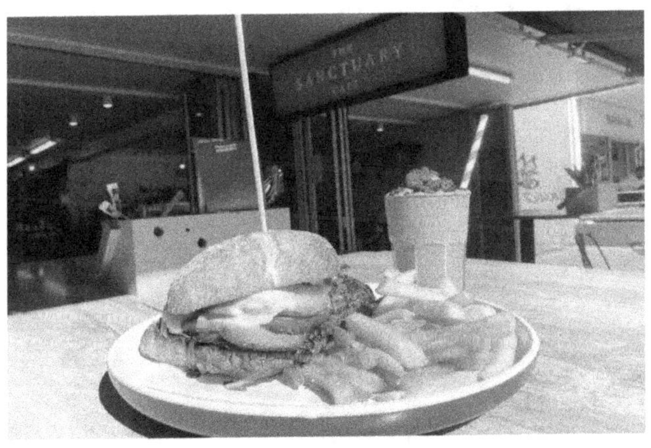

Dayna G. Murphy

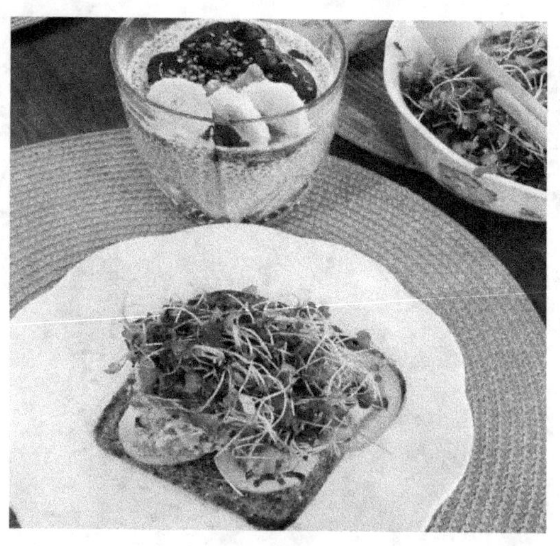

Table of Contents

INTRODUCTION

The Blood Type O Cookbook is a simple and delicious guide to eating appropriately for your blood type. If you're type O, this cookbook is designed specifically for you, with simple dishes that meet your specific requirements. Eating the appropriate meals can have a major impact on how you feel, and this cookbook can help. It is jam-packed with delicious meals and snacks, making it easy to select the proper ingredients. Each recipe, from hearty breakfasts to filling feasts, is designed with your health in mind. You'll discover the power of foods that are compatible with your blood type, boosting healthy digestion, energy, and weight management. Prepare to start on a tasty journey toward better health and vitality with the Blood Type O Cookbook, since eating properly should be simple and pleasurable.

CHAPTER 1

Understanding Blood Type O

What Exactly Is the Blood Type O Diet?

The Blood Type O diet is a dietary plan that is based on the premise that a person's blood type influences their nutritional demands and how their body processes food. According to a naturopathic physician idea, people with blood type O have different nutritional needs than those with other blood types (A, B, or AB).

Healthy Foods

Certain meals are recommended for blood type O individuals because they are thought to accord with their genetic composition and provide optimal health advantages. The following foods should be included in the Blood Type O diet:

Proteins that are low in fat:

- Grass-fed beef, lamb, and poultry are examples of lean meats.
- Salmon, mackerel, and cod are examples of cold-water fish.
- Venison and buffalo are examples of wild game.

Vegetables and fruits:

- Kale, spinach, and collard greens are examples of dark leafy greens.
- Blueberries, strawberries, and blackberries, in particular.
- Sweet potatoes and carrots are examples of root vegetables.
- Broccoli and cauliflower are examples of cruciferous veggies.

Dairy and Dairy Substitutes:

- Goat cheese with goat milk.
- Almond milk and rice milk are dairy replacements.

Grains:

- Quinoa and amaranth are ancient cereals.
- Rice, particularly brown and wild rice.

Seeds and nuts:

- Walnuts, flaxseeds, and pumpkin seeds are all good sources of omega-3 fatty acids.

Fats that are good for you:

- Flaxseed oil and olive oil.

Seasonings and spices:

- Turmeric, ginger, and garlic.

- The salt from the sea.

Foods to Stay Away From

The Blood Type O diet suggests avoiding or limiting some foods that may not be well tolerated by people with blood type O. Foods to avoid in general include:

Milk and dairy products:

- Cheese and cow's milk.
- Ice cream and butter.

Grains:

- Wheat goods such as bread and pasta.
- Rye and barley.

Legumes:

- Avoid or limit your consumption of legumes such as lentils, kidney beans, and peanuts.

Specific Fruits:

- Oranges and strawberries should be consumed in moderation.

Sugary and processed foods:

- Processed and high-sugar foods should be avoided.

Black tea with coffee:

- Limit your intake of coffee and black tea.

Meats that have been highly processed:

- Meats that have been processed, such as bacon and sausage.

The Advantages of Eating for Your Blood Type

Proponents of the Blood Type O diet argue that eating according to your blood type can provide a variety of benefits, including:

1. Improved Digestion: Eating meals that are appropriate for your blood type may result in better digestion and less gastrointestinal discomfort.

2. Enhanced Energy Levels: The diet is designed to give nutrients that can assist raise energy and vitality, resulting in increased stamina and overall performance.

3. Adherence to the diet may aid in weight control attempts and the maintenance of a healthy body weight.

4. Better Immune Function: According to some proponents, eating according to your blood type may enhance your immune system, thereby lowering your risk of certain illnesses.

5. Inflammation can be reduced by avoiding foods that are incompatible with your blood type.

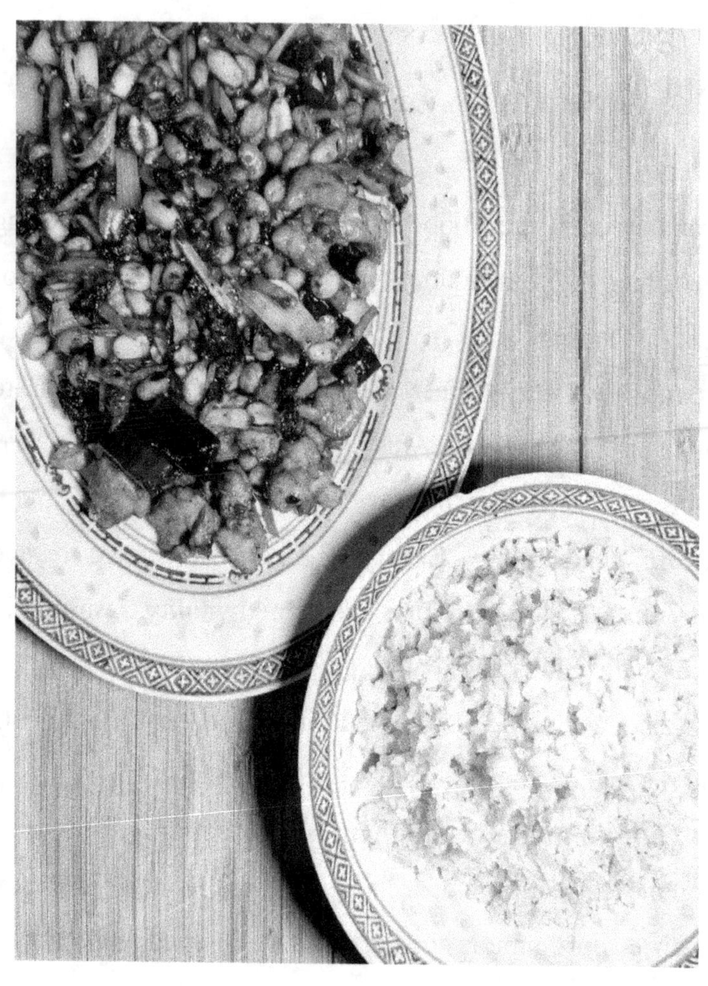

CHAPTER 2

BLOOD TYPE O RECOMMENDED FOODS

1. MEAT AND POULTRY

Meat/Poultry	Portion Size	Frequency per Week
Grass-fed Beef	4-6 ounces	3-4 times per week
Lamb	4-6 ounces	2-3 times per week
Poultry (Chicken, Turkey)	4-6 ounces	3-4 times per week
Wild Game (Venison, Buffalo)	4-6 ounces	1-2 times per week
Cold-Water Fish (Salmon,	6 ounces	2-3 times per week

| Mackerel, Cod) | | |

2. DIARY AND EGGS

Dairy/Eggs	Portion Size	Frequency per Week
Goat's Milk	1 cup	3-4 times per week
Goat Cheese	1-2 ounces	2-3 times per week
Almond Milk	1 cup	3-4 times per week
Rice Milk	1 cup	3-4 times per week
Eggs	2-3 eggs	3-4 times per week

3. SEAFOODS

Seafood	Portion Size	Frequency per Week
Salmon	4-6 ounces	2-3 times per week
Mackerel	4-6 ounces	2-3 times per week
Cod	4-6 ounces	2-3 times per week
Sardines	4-6 ounces	1-2 times per week
Trout	4-6 ounces	2-3 times per week
Halibut	4-6 ounces	2-3 times per week

4. NUTS AND SEEDS

Nuts/Seeds	Portion Size	Frequency per Week

Walnuts	1/4 cup	3-4 times per week
Flaxseeds	1 tablespoon	3-4 times per week
Pumpkin Seeds	1/4 cup	2-3 times per week
Chia Seeds	1 tablespoon	2-3 times per week
Almonds	1/4 cup	3-4 times per week
Sunflower Seeds	1/4 cup	2-3 times per week
Pecans	1/4 cup	2-3 times per week

5. GRAINS AND CEREALS

Grains/Cereals	Portion Size	Frequency per Week

Quinoa	1/2 cup (cooked)	3-4 times per week
Amaranth	1/2 cup (cooked)	2-3 times per week
Brown Rice	1/2 cup (cooked)	3-4 times per week
Wild Rice	1/2 cup (cooked)	2-3 times per week
Oats (Steel-Cut or Rolled)	1/2 cup (cooked)	2-3 times per week
Buckwheat	1/2 cup (cooked)	2-3 times per week
Millet	1/2 cup (cooked)	2-3 times per week

6. BEVERAGES, TEAS AND COFFEE

Beverages	Portion Size	Frequency per Week
Water	8 ounces	Daily

Green Tea	1 cup	3-4 times per week
Herbal Tea (e.g., Peppermint, Ginger)	1 cup	2-3 times per week
Rooibos Tea	1 cup	2-3 times per week
Dandelion Tea	1 cup	2-3 times per week
Black Tea (limited)	1 cup	1-2 times per week
Coffee (limited)	8 ounces	1-2 times per week

7. FRUITS

Fruits	Portion Size	Frequency per Week
Berries (Blueberries,	1/2 cup	3-4 times per week

Strawberries, Blackberries)		
Cherries	1/2 cup	2-3 times per week
Pineapple	1/2 cup (fresh)	2-3 times per week
Plums	1 medium	2-3 times per week
Papaya	1/2 cup (fresh)	2-3 times per week
Figs	2 medium	1-2 times per week
Prunes	2-3 pieces	1-2 times per week

8. HERBS AND SPICES

Herbs/Spices	Portion Size	Frequency per Week

Ginger	1 teaspoon	3-4 times per week
Garlic	1-2 cloves	3-4 times per week
Turmeric	1/2 teaspoon	2-3 times per week
Thyme	1 teaspoon	2-3 times per week
Rosemary	1 teaspoon	2-3 times per week
Basil	1 tablespoon	2-3 times per week
Oregano	1 teaspoon	2-3 times per week
Sea Salt	As needed	As needed

9. VEGETABLES

Vegetables	Portion Size	Frequency per Week

Dark Leafy Greens (Kale, Spinach, Collard Greens)	1 cup	4-5 times per week
Broccoli	1/2 cup (cooked)	3-4 times per week
Cauliflower	1/2 cup (cooked)	3-4 times per week
Sweet Potatoes	1 medium	3-4 times per week
Carrots	1 medium	2-3 times per week
Beetroot	1/2 cup (cooked)	2-3 times per week
Onions	1/2 cup (cooked)	2-3 times per week
Garlic	1-2 cloves	3-4 times per week

10. BEANS AND LEGUMES

Beans/Legumes	Portion Size	Frequency per Week
Black-Eyed Peas	1/2 cup (cooked)	1-2 times per week
Lentils	1/2 cup (cooked)	1-2 times per week
Adzuki Beans	1/2 cup (cooked)	1-2 times per week
Pinto Beans	1/2 cup (cooked)	1-2 times per week
Navy Beans	1/2 cup (cooked)	1-2 times per week

11. OILS AND FATS

Oils/Fats	Portion Size	Frequency per Week
Olive Oil	1 tablespoon	Daily

Flaxseed Oil	1 teaspoon	3-4 times per week
Walnut Oil	1 teaspoon	2-3 times per week
Coconut Oil	1 teaspoon	1-2 times per week
Ghee (Clarified Butter)	1 teaspoon	2-3 times per week
Avocado	1/4 to 1/2 avocado	3-4 times per week
Nuts (Almonds, Walnuts)	1/4 cup	3-4 times per week
Seeds (Chia, Flaxseeds)	1 tablespoon	3-4 times per week

CHAPTER 3

RECIPES AND INGREDIENTS

10 BREAKFAST DELIGHTS

ENERGIZING OMELETTE

Ingredients

- 3 big eggs
- 1/4 cup diced turkey
- 14 cup diced bell peppers

Instructions:

1. Season with salt and pepper to taste
2. In a bowl, whisk together the eggs and season with salt and pepper.
3. Sauté the turkey, spinach, and bell peppers in a nonstick skillet until done.
4. Pour the whisked eggs over the ingredients and simmer until set.
5. Fold the omelette in half and serve.

SPICED SWEET POTATO PANCAKES

Ingredients

- 1 cup shredded sweet potatoes
- 2 eggs
- 2 tbsp almond flour
- 1/2 teaspoon cinnamon
- 1/4 teaspoon nutmeg

Instructions:

1. In a bowl, combine all of the ingredients.
2. Warm a skillet and put pieces of the mixture into it.
3. Cook until the edges are golden brown, then turn and cook the other side.
4. Serve with a dollop of Greek yogurt.

SMOOTHIE WITH NUT BUTTER AND BANANAS

Ingredients

- 1 banana
- 1 tbsp almond butter
- 1/2 cup almond milk
- Ice cubes (optional)

Instructions:

1. Blend banana, almond butter, and almond milk until smooth.
2. If desired, add ice cubes and mix one more.
3. Pour into a glass and serve.

FRUIT-FILLED QUINOA BOWL

Ingredients

- 1/2 cup cooked quinoa
- 1/2 cup mixed berries (blueberries, strawberries)
- 1 tablespoon chopped walnuts
- 1 tbsp flaxseeds

Instructions:

1. In a mixing bowl, combine the cooked quinoa, berries, walnuts, and flaxseeds.
2. Mix well and serve.

BAKED SWEET POTATO FRIES WITH EGGS

Ingredients

- 1 sweet potato, cut into fries
- 2 eggs
- 1 tbsp olive oil

Instructions:

1. Toss sweet potato fries in olive oil, salt, and pepper to taste.
2. Bake till crispy.
3. Cook the eggs as desired and serve with the sweet potato fries.

QUINOA-STUFFED BELL PEPPERS

Ingredients

- 2 bell peppers, halves and seeds removed
- 1/2 cup cooked quinoa
- 1/4 cup chopped tomatoes
- 1/4 cup drained and rinsed black beans

Instructions:

1. Preheat the oven to 375°F (190°C).
2. In a mixing bowl, combine the quinoa, diced tomatoes, and black beans.
3. Stuff bell pepper halves with the quinoa mixture.
4. Bake until the peppers are soft.

BERRY CHIA SEED PUDDING

Ingredients

- 2 tbsp chia seeds
- 1/2 cup almond milk
- berries for decoration

Instructions:

1. In a jar, combine the chia seeds and almond milk.
2. Refrigerate overnight.
3. Before serving, garnish with mixed berries.

CREAMY AVOCADO AND CUCUMBER SOUP

Ingredients

- 1 ripe avocado
- 1 cucumber, peeled and diced
- 1 cup plain Greek yogurt
- 1/2 cup water

Instructions:

1. Blend avocado, cucumber, Greek yogurt, and water until smooth.
2. Refrigerate before serving.

MIXED BERRY SMOOTHIE

Ingredients

- 1 cup mixed berries (strawberries, blueberries, raspberries) 1/2 banana
- 1/2 cup almond milk
- Toppings: sliced almonds, chia seeds

Instructions:

1. Blend the mixed berries, banana, and almond milk until smooth.
2. Place in a bowl and top with desired toppings.

SPICED SWEET POTATO HASH

Ingredients

- 1 sweet potato, grated
- 1/4 cup diced turkey or chicken
- 1/4 cup diced onions
- 1/2 teaspoon paprika

Instructions:

1. Cook sweet potato, turkey, and onions in a pan until done.
2. Season with paprika and cook until flavors combine.

These recipes include a combination of savory and sweet options, giving variety for some blood type O's breakfast preferences. Prep times vary, but most of these recipes may be made in 20-30 minutes. Individual preferences and dietary demands should be taken into account when adjusting quantities and ingredients. Enjoy!

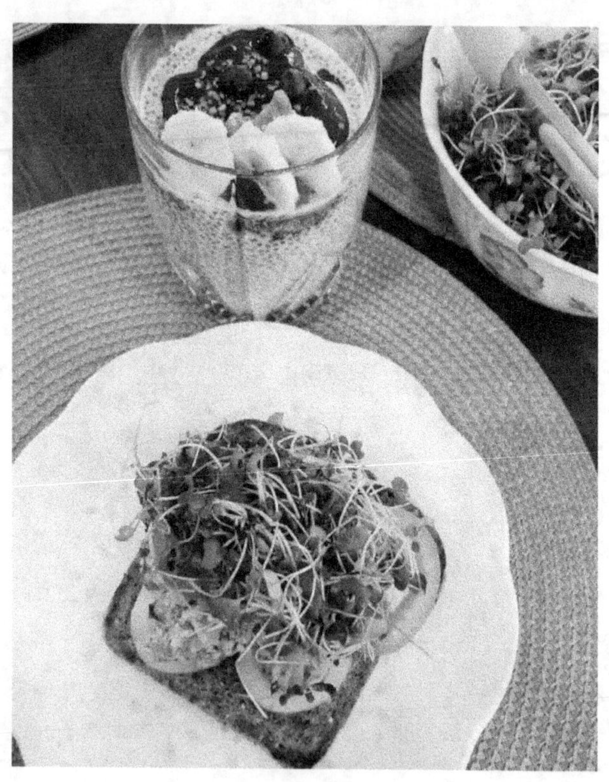

GRILLED SALMON SALAD

Ingredients

- 6 oz. grilled salmon
- Greens (kale and spinach)
- Cherry tomatoes, cucumber halves, sliced olive oil, and lemon dressing

Instructions:

1. Grill the fish until it is done.
2. Combine mixed greens, cherry tomatoes, and cucumber in a salad bowl.
3. Drizzle with olive oil and lemon dressing and top with grilled fish.

Preparation Time: 20 minutes

STUFFED BELL PEPPERS WITH QUINOA

Ingredients

- 2 bell peppers, cut in half and seeds removed
- 1 cooked cup quinoa
- a quarter cup chopped tomatoes
- 1/4 cup washed and drained black beans

Instructions:

1. Preheat the oven to 375 degrees Fahrenheit (190 degrees Celsius).
2. In a mixing bowl, combine quinoa, chopped tomatoes, and black beans.
3. Stuff the quinoa mixture into the bell pepper halves.
4. Bake until the peppers are soft.

Preparation Time: 30 minutes

TURKEY AND LENTIL SOUP

Ingredients

- 1/2 cup cooked lentils
- 1/2 cup turkey, diced
- Diced carrots, celery, and onions
- Broth (chicken or veggie)

Instructions:

1. In a pot, sauté the turkey, carrots, celery, and onions.
2. Pour in the cooked lentils and broth.
3. Cook until the vegetables are soft.

Preparation Time: 25 minutes

ZUCCHINI NOODLES WITH PESTO AND CHERRY TOMATOES

Ingredients

- Zucchini noodle soup
- Pesto sauce (basil, pine nuts, and olive oil)
- halved cherry tomatoes
- Optional: grated Parmesan cheese

Instructions:

1. Make zucchini noodles by spiralizing it.
2. Combine pesto sauce and cherry tomatoes in a mixing bowl.
3. If desired, sprinkle with Parmesan cheese.

Preparation Time: 15 minutes

STIR-FRY WITH CHICKEN AND VEGETABLES

Ingredients

- 4 ounces grilled chicken, thinly sliced
- Florets of broccoli
- Snow peas, sliced bell peppers
- Soy sauce, ginger, and garlic stir-fry sauce

Instructions:

1. In a pan, stir-fry the chicken and veggies.
2. Cook until the stir-fry sauce is cooked thoroughly.
3. Over brown rice or quinoa, serve.

Preparation Time: 20 minutes

MASHED SWEET POTATOES WITH TURKEY PATTIES

Ingredients

- 1 medium sweet potato, mashed
- Turkey patties
- Green beans, steamed

Instructions:

1. Cook turkey patties according per package directions.
2. Steam green beans and mash sweet potatoes.
3. Serve the turkey patties atop mashed sweet potatoes with green beans on the side.

Preparation Time: 25 minutes

ROASTED ASPARAGUS WITH LEMON ZEST

Ingredients

- fresh asparagus spears
- Extra virgin olive oil
- Zest of lemon
- a pinch of sea salt

Instructions:

1. Preheat the oven to 400 degrees Fahrenheit (200 degrees Celsius).
2. Roast the asparagus in olive oil until tender.
3. Season with lemon zest and sea salt to taste.

Preparation Time: 15 minutes

RED LENTIL AND SPINACH CURRY

Ingredients

- 1/2 cup cooked red lentils
- Spinach stems
- Coconut cream
- Curry spices (turmeric, cumin, coriander)

Instructions:

1. In a pan, sauté spinach until wilted.
2. Cooked red lentils, coconut milk, and curry spices are added.
3. Simmer until the flavors blend.
4. Over brown rice, serve.

Preparation Time: 30 minutes

HUMMUS AND CELERY STACKS

Ingredients

- celery sticks
- Hummus
- halved cherry tomatoes
- Cucumber slices

Instructions:

1. Spread hummus on celery sticks and serve.
2. Serve with cherry tomatoes and cucumber slices on top.

Preparation Time: 10 minutes

SALAD WITH BEETS AND SPINACH WITH ALMONDS

Ingredients

- Roasted and sliced beets
- spinach leaves, fresh
- Almonds, sliced
- Dressing: balsamic vinaigrette

Instructions:

1. Beets should be roasted and sliced.
2. Toss spinach with beets and almond slices.
3. Drizzle with balsamic vinaigrette and serve.

Preparation Time: 25 minutes

GRILLED CHICKEN WITH BROCCOLI AND QUINOA

Ingredients

- 1 6 oz. grilled chicken breast
- 1 cup broccoli, steaming
- 1 cooked cup quinoa
- Seasonings include olive oil, lemon, and herbs

Instructions:

1. Grill the chicken until done, then season with olive oil, lemon, and herbs.
2. Separately, steam the broccoli and cook the quinoa.
3. Serve grilled chicken over quinoa with steamed broccoli on the side.

Preparation Time: 30 minutes

SHRIMP STIR-FRIED WITH VEGETABLES

Ingredients

- 8 ounces peeled and deveined shrimp
- Vegetable mixture (bell peppers, broccoli, snow peas)
- Garlic and ginger for flavor
- Soy sauce or tamari

Instructions:

1. Stir-fry the shrimp and vegetables with the ginger and garlic.
2. Season with tamari or soy sauce.
3. Over brown rice, serve.

Preparation Time: 25 minutes

SALMON BAKED WITH ROASTED VEGETABLES

Ingredients

- 6 oz. salmon fillet
- Vegetables (zucchini, cherry tomatoes, and bell peppers)
- Seasonings include olive oil, lemon, and dill.

Instructions:

1. Preheat the oven to 400 degrees Fahrenheit (200 degrees Celsius).
2. Place the salmon on a baking sheet, surrounded by the veggies, and season with olive oil, lemon juice, and dill.
3. Bake until the fish is done and the veggies are roasted.

Preparation Time: 30 minutes

SKEWERS OF TURKEY AND VEGETABLES

Ingredients

- chunks of turkey
- Tomatoes in the shape of cherries
- Red onion, sliced bell peppers, chunked
- Marinade with olive oil and herbs

Instructions:

1. Marinate turkey cubes in olive oil and herbs for 30 minutes.
2. Thread skewers with turkey, tomatoes, onion, and bell peppers.
3. Grill until the turkey is cooked through and the vegetables are soft.

Preparation Time: 25 minutes

EGGPLANT AND CHICKPEA CURRY

Ingredients

- 1 large chopped eggplant 1 can drained and rinsed chickpeas Tomatoes, diced
- Curry spices (cumin, coriander, turmeric) Sauté the eggplant till golden.

Instructions:

1. Mix in the chickpeas, tomatoes, and curry spices.
2. Simmer until the flavors blend.
3. Over brown rice, serve.

Preparation Time: 30 minutes

TURKEY AND SWEET POTATO HASH

Ingredients

- ground turkey
- Sweet potatoes, onion, garlic, and chopped parsley
- Seasonings: paprika and cayenne pepper

Instructions:

1. In a pan, sauté the turkey, sweet potatoes, onion, and garlic.
2. Paprika and cayenne pepper to taste.
3. Cook until the turkey is browned and the sweet potatoes are soft.

Preparation Time: 25 minutes

BAKED LEMON HERB CHICKEN THIGHS

Ingredients

- ground turkey
- Sweet potatoes, onion, garlic, and chopped parsley
- Seasonings: paprika and cayenne pepper
- Chicken thighs are the main ingredients.
- Juice of lemon
- Herbs (rosemary and thyme)
- sliced garlic

Instructions:

1. Preheat the oven to 375 degrees Fahrenheit (190 degrees Celsius).
2. In a baking dish, place the chicken thighs.
3. Drizzle with lemon juice and top with fresh herbs and garlic minced.
4. Bake until the chicken is thoroughly done.

Preparation Time: 35 minutes

GROUND BEEF STUFFED BELL PEPPERS

Ingredients

- half bell peppers with seeds removed
- seasoned ground beef
- Quinoa
- Tomatoes and onions, diced

Instructions:

1. Brown the ground beef, then combine it with the cooked quinoa, diced tomatoes, and onions.
2. Stuff bell pepper halves with the mixture and bake until soft.

Preparation Time: 40 minutes

MUSHROOM AND SPINACH OMELETTE

Ingredients

- 3 eggs
- Mushrooms, cut
- Spinach stems
- Optional goat cheese

Instructions:

1. Whisk the eggs and throw them into a hot skillet.
2. Mix in the mushrooms and spinach.
3. Cook until the eggs are firm, then fold in half and top with goat cheese if preferred.

Preparation Time: 15 minutes

CAULIFLOWER FRIED RICE WITH SHRIMP

Ingredients

- Rice made from cauliflower
- Peeled and deveined shrimp
- Vegetables (peas, carrots, and corn)
- Seasonings: soy sauce and ginger

Instructions:

1. Sauté shrimp and mixed vegetables in a skillet.
2. Stir in the cauliflower rice.
3. Season with soy sauce and ginger to taste.

Preparation Time: 25 minutes

GUACAMOLE WITH VEGETABLE STICKS

Ingredients

- 12 ripe avocados are used in this recipe.
- Juice of lime
- sliced garlic
- Cherry tomatoes, carrot dice, and cucumber sticks

Instructions:

1. Mash avocados and combine with lime juice, minced garlic, and diced tomatoes.
2. Serve with cucumber and carrot sticks.

Preparation Time: 10 minutes

GREEK YOGURT AND BERRY PARFAIT

Ingredients

- Greek yogurt
- Mixed berries (strawberries, blueberries)
- sliced honey almonds

Instructions:

1. In a glass, combine Greek yogurt and mixed berries.
2. Drizzle with honey and sprinkle with almond slices.

Preparation Time: 5 minutes

CUCUMBER AND SMOKED SALMON BITES

Ingredients

- Cucumber slices
- Salmon smoked
- The cream cheeses

Instructions:

1. Arrange cucumber slices on a plate and top with smoked salmon and a small dollop of cream cheese.
2. Garnish with dill, if desired.

Preparation Time: 15 minutes

ROASTED CHICKPEAS

Ingredients

- drained and rinsed canned chickpeas
- Olive oil
- Cumin and paprika

Instructions:

1. Toss the chickpeas with the olive oil, paprika, and cumin.
2. Roast till crispy in the oven.

Preparation Time: 30 minutes

KALE CHIPS

Ingredients

- Torn fresh kale leaves into bite-sized pieces
- Extra virgin olive oil
- Sea salt

Instructions:

1. Massage kale leaves with olive oil and sprinkle with sea salt.
2. Bake until the bacon is crispy.

Preparation Time: 20 minutes

STUFFED MUSHROOMS WITH GOAT CHEESE

Ingredients

- cleaned mushrooms with stems removed
- The goat cheese
- sliced garlic
- fresh herbs (thyme, rosemary)

Instructions:

1. Combine goat cheese, minced garlic, and fresh herbs in a mixing bowl.
2. Fill the mushrooms with the mixture.
3. Bake until the mushrooms are soft.

Preparation Time: 25 minutes.

ALMOND BUTTER APPLE SLICES

Ingredients

- apple, sliced
- almond butter
- Optional cinnamon

Instructions:

1. Spread almond butter on apple slices and serve.
2. If desired, sprinkle with cinnamon.

Preparation Time: 5 minutes

BRUSCHETTA TOMATO BASIL

Ingredients

- chopped tomatoes
- fresh basil, chopped
- minced garlic
- Extra virgin olive oil
- Baguette slices, whole grain or gluten-free

Instructions:

1. Mix tomatoes, basil, and minced garlic together.
2. Allow to marinate after drizzling with olive oil.
3. Serve with slices of toasted baguette.

Preparation Time: 15 minutes

SPICY ROASTED ALMONDS

Ingredients

- Almonds
- Extra virgin olive oil
- Chili powder
- a pinch of sea salt

Instructions:

1. Toss the almonds with the olive oil, cayenne pepper, and sea salt.
2. Roast until golden and aromatic.

Preparation Time: 15 minutes

CAPRESE SKEWERS

Ingredients

- cherry tomatoes
- Balls of mozzarella
- Basil leaves, fresh
- Glazed with balsamic vinegar

Instructions:

1. Thread cherry tomatoes, mozzarella balls, and basil leaves onto skewers and serve.
2. Before serving, drizzle with balsamic glaze.

Preparation Time: 10 minutes

MIXED BERRY CHIA SEED PUDDING

Ingredients

- 2 teaspoons chia seeds

- a half-cup almond milk

- Mixed berries (strawberries, blueberries)

- For sweetness, use honey or maple syrup.

Instructions:

1. In a jar, combine chia seeds and almond milk.

2. Refrigerate for at least 24 hours.

3. Before serving, top with mixed berries and drizzle with honey or maple syrup.

Time to prepare: 10 minutes (+ overnight refrigerated)

DARK CHOCOLATE-DIPPED STRAWBERRIES

Ingredients

- fresh strawberries
- Melted dark chocolate

Instructions:

1. Dip each strawberry into the melted dark chocolate.
2. Place on a tray lined with parchment paper.
3. Before serving, allow the chocolate to set.

Preparation Time: 20 minutes

ALMOND FLOUR BANANA MUFFINS

Ingredients

- 2 ripe bananas, mashed
- 2 tbsp almond flour
- 3 eggs
- 1 tablespoon coconut oil
- Baking soda

Instructions:

1. Preheat the oven to 350 degrees Fahrenheit (175 degrees Celsius).
2. Mash bananas, almond flour, eggs, coconut oil, and baking powder together.
3. Fill muffin cups halfway with batter and bake until golden.

Preparation Time: 25 minutes

COCONUT YOGURT

Ingredients

- Berries (raspberries and blackberries)
- shred coconut

Instructions:

1. In a glass, combine coconut yogurt and mixed berries.
2. Finish with shredded coconut.

Preparation Time: 10 minutes

CINNAMON BAKED APPLE

Ingredients

- Apple, cored
- sliced Cinnamon Honey (optional)

Instructions:

1. Preheat the oven to 375 degrees Fahrenheit (190 degrees Celsius).
2. Arrange the apple slices on a baking pan.
3. Sprinkle with cinnamon and bake until the potatoes are soft.
4. If desired, drizzle with honey.

Preparation Time: 15 minutes.

SORBET PINEAPPLE COCONUT

Ingredients

- Fresh pineapple and coconut milk, diced
- Juice of lime
- For sweetness, use honey or agave syrup.

Instructions:

1. Blend the pineapple, coconut milk, lime juice, and sweetener till smooth.
2. Pour into a plate and place in the freezer until hard.
3. Scoop and plate.

Preparation Time: 15 minutes. (plus freezing time)

MOUSSE AVOCADO CHOCOLATE

Ingredients

- Avocados that are ripe

- cacao powder

- Agar nectar or maple syrup

- Vanilla flavoring

Instructions:

1. Blend avocados. Cocoa powder, sweetner, and vanilla until smooth

2. Chill in the refrigerator before serving

Preparation Time: 10 minutes).

ENERGY BITES WITH WALNUTS AND DATES

Ingredients

- Walnuts are one of the ingredients.
- pitted dates
- toasted coconut flakes
- Vanilla extract

Instructions:

1. In a food processor, combine walnuts, dates, coconut flakes, and vanilla.
2. Make bite-sized balls out of the dough.
3. Allow to cool before serving.

Preparation Time: 15 minutes

PEAR BAKED WITH CINNAMON AND ALMONDS

Ingredients

- Ripe pear, cut in half and cored
- Cinnamon
- Almonds, sliced

Instructions:

- Preheat the oven to 375 degrees Fahrenheit (190 degrees Celsius).
- Arrange the pear halves on a baking sheet.
- Garnish with cinnamon and chopped almonds.
- Bake until the potatoes are soft.

Preparation Time: 20 minutes

CHERRY ALMOND SMOOTHIE BOWL

Ingredients

- Frozen cherries
- Milk made from almonds
- The almond butter
- Toppings include sliced almonds and shredded coconut.

Instructions:

Blend the frozen cherries, almond milk, and almond butter until creamy.

Pour into a bowl and top with desired toppings.

Preparation Time: 10 minutes

BERRY BLAST SMOOTHIE

Ingredients

- 1 cup mixed berries (blueberries, strawberries, raspberries)
- a half banana
- a half-cup almond milk
- 1 teaspoon chia seeds
- Cubes of ice

Instructions:

1. Blend the berries, banana, almond milk, and chia seeds until smooth.
2. Blend in the ice cubes again.

Preparation Time: 5 minutes

GREEN TROPICAL SMOOTHIE

Ingredients

- 1 cup fresh spinach leaves
- 1 pound pineapple chunks
- a half banana
- 1 cup of coconut water
- 1 teaspoon flaxseed

Instructions:

1. Blend spinach, pineapple, banana, coconut water, and flaxseeds together until smooth.

Preparation Time: 5 minutes

AVOCADO AND KALE DELIGHT

Ingredients

- 1/2 avocado
- 1 cup kale leaves, trimmed
- 1/2 cup sliced cucumber
- a half-cup almond milk
- 1 heaping tablespoon hemp seeds

Instructions:

1. Blend avocado, kale, cucumber, almond milk, and hemp seeds together until smooth.

Preparation Time: 5 minutes

BANANA ALMOND BUTTER SMOOTHIE

Ingredients

- 1 banana
- two tbsp almond butter
- 1/2 cup plain Greek yogurt
- a half-cup almond milk
- Cubes of ice

Instructions:

1. Blend the banana, almond butter, Greek yogurt, and almond milk together until smooth.
2. Blend in the ice cubes again.

Preparation Time: 5 minutes

PINEAPPLE MINT COOLER

Ingredients

- 1 cup pineapple chunks

- a few fresh mint leaves

- 1/2 cucumber, cut 1/2 lime, lime juice

Instructions:

1. Blend pineapple, mint leaves, cucumber, lime juice, and coconut water together until smooth.

Preparation Time: 5 minutes

CHERRY ALMOND SMOOTHIE

Ingredients

- 1 cup frozen cherries
- a half-cup almond milk
- a quarter cup almonds
- 1 banana, 1 cup Greek yogurt

Instructions:

1. Blend frozen cherries, almond milk, almonds, banana, and Greek yogurt together until smooth.

Preparation Time: 5 minutes

SMOOTHIE WITH MANGO, SPINACH, AND SUNSHINE

Ingredients

- 1 cup mango pieces
- a few of spinach leaves
- half a cup orange juice
- Chia seeds and half a banana

Instructions:

1. Mango, spinach, orange juice, banana, and chia seeds should be blended until smooth.

Preparation Time: 5 minutes

SMOOTHIE WITH COCOA BANANA PROTEIN

Ingredients

- 1 banana is used as an ingredient.
- 1 teaspoon cocoa powder
- 1/2 cup plain Greek yogurt
- a half-cup almond milk
- Optional protein powder

Instructions:

1. Blend banana, cocoa powder, Greek yogurt, almond milk, and protein powder together until smooth.

Preparation Time: 5 minutes

STRAWBERRY COCONUT DREAM

Ingredients

- 1 cup strawberries
- a half-cup coconut milk
- a half banana
- 1 tbsp. shredded coconut
- Cubes of ice

Instructions:

1. Strawberries, coconut milk, banana, shredded coconut, and ice cubes should be blended until smooth.

Preparation Time: 5 minutes

BLUEBERRY BLISS SMOOTHIE

Ingredients

- 1 cup blueberries
- 1/2 cup plain Greek yogurt
- a half-cup almond milk
- 1 teaspoon chia seeds
- Honey is used to add sweetness.

Instructions:

2. Blend blueberries, greek yoghurt, almond milk, chia seeds, and honey until smooth.

Preparation Time: 5 minutes

CONCLUSION

Finally, the Blood Type O Cookbook is your guide to a nutritious diet made exclusively for people with blood type O. It is filled with delicious recipes and emphasizes the importance of eating foods that are appropriate for blood type O. The cookbook recommends meal sizes and weekly frequency to promote well-being. It empowers blood type O persons to make informed choices for improved digestion, energy levels, and weight control by including appropriate meats, seafood, fruits, and vegetables.

The cookbook transforms dining into a conscious experience, strengthening the link between nutrition and personal health. It includes recipes for every meal, from nutritious breakfasts to filling meals and guilt-free treats. **The Blood Type O Cookbook**, with its simplicity and flavor, urges people to embrace a healthier lifestyle adapted to their blood type, turning the journey to vitality into a joyful culinary adventure.

7 DAYS MEAL PLAN

Day 1:

Breakfast: Berry Blast Smoothie (Mixed berries, banana, almond milk, chia seeds)

Lunch: Grilled Chicken Salad (Mixed greens, cherry tomatoes, grilled chicken, olive oil dressing)

Dinner: Baked Salmon with Roasted Vegetables (Salmon fillet, zucchini, cherry tomatoes, olive oil, lemon, dill)

Day 2:

Breakfast: Avocado and Kale Delight Smoothie (Avocado, kale, cucumber, almond milk, hemp seeds)

Lunch: Quinoa-Stuffed Bell Peppers (Quinoa, diced tomatoes, black beans, bell peppers)

Dinner: Stir-Fried Shrimp with Vegetables (Shrimp, bell peppers, broccoli, snow peas, tamari sauce)

Day 3:

Breakfast: Green Tropical Smoothie (Spinach, pineapple, banana, coconut water, flaxseeds)

Lunch: Turkey and Lentil Soup (Cooked lentils, diced turkey, carrots, celery, onions)

Dinner: Eggplant and Chickpea Curry (Eggplant, chickpeas, tomatoes, curry spices)

Day 4:

Breakfast: Banana Almond Butter Smoothie (Banana, almond butter, Greek yogurt, almond milk)

Lunch: Zucchini Noodles with Pesto and Cherry Tomatoes (Zucchini noodles, pesto sauce, cherry tomatoes)

Dinner: Baked Chicken with Broccoli and Quinoa (Grilled chicken, steamed broccoli, cooked quinoa)

Day 5:

Breakfast: Cocoa Banana Protein Smoothie (Banana, cocoa powder, Greek yogurt, almond milk, protein powder)

Lunch: Chicken and Vegetable Stir-Fry (Grilled chicken, broccoli, bell peppers, snow peas, stir-fry sauce)

Dinner: Mushroom and Spinach Omelette (Eggs, mushrooms, spinach, goat cheese)

Day 6:

Breakfast: Pineapple Mint Cooler Smoothie (Pineapple chunks, mint leaves, cucumber, lime juice, coconut water)

Lunch: Hummus and Celery Stacks (Celery sticks, hummus, cherry tomatoes, sliced cucumbers)

Dinner: Turkey and Sweet Potato Hash (Ground turkey, sweet potatoes, onion, garlic, paprika, cayenne pepper)

Day 7:

Breakfast: Blueberry Bliss Smoothie (Blueberries, Greek yogurt, almond milk, chia seeds, honey)

Lunch: Caprese Skewers (Cherry tomatoes, mozzarella balls, fresh basil leaves, balsamic glaze)

Dinner: Stuffed Bell Peppers with Ground Beef (Ground beef, quinoa, diced tomatoes, onions)

Adjust portion sizes based on individual needs, and feel free to swap recipes to suit personal preferences. Remember to stay hydrated and listen to your body throughout the week. Enjoy your delicious and nourishing meals!

HAPPY

COOKING!